A MUSLIMAH'S GUIDE TO

Healthy
Hijab Hair

JENNIFER OGUNYEMI

First Edition, 2018

Copyright 2018 A Muslimah's Guide to Healthy Afro Hijab Hair

Written by Jennifer Ogynyemi

Layout by Reyhana Ismail: www.reyoflightdesign.com

Dedication

I would like to dedicate this book to my girls Amaara and Amaya for giving me the inspiration and vision to write this book.

To my boys:
Abdul Maalik for being patient with me as I constantly bother him to read through every page and had already bought a book before it being published.

Dayyaan for being the first person to hear me scream at seeing this book come to into exisistence.

My husband, you are my rock, motivation and my accountability partner. You have watched me grow and evolve whilst guiding me through this life we have built together, you have allowed me to bother you with my ideas and screaming at me to write them down. Alhamdulillah I listened this time.

Lastly to myself to showing my worth, my strength and self love.

Introduction

Asalaamu alaikum, my dear sister.

I pray this book reaches you and your hair in a state that is well and healthy.

Since covering your hair with hijab, have you found yourself struggling with your hair care?

Maybe you have abandoned your relaxed hair out of fear of losing it to the constant battle of getting it wet. Or it could be that you have given up on your natural tresses because you have told yourself your hair is just too difficult to deal with under wraps.

Sister, whatever your hair struggles are, you are not alone.

This book will teach you techniques that can be used by even the busiest of ladies, insha'Allah; tips that will allow you to manage your hair faster and easier, and cheats for wives and wives-to-be who need a quick-fix to having better hair days and nights.
You are the reason why I wrote this little guide. I, too, went through a

phase of being unsure of what to do and how to do with the little time I had as a wife and mother. As a hair care stylist and being on a healthy hair journey of my own, I have compiled all the issues we face as women with beautiful kinks in our hair, and provided solutions as well as how we can deal with them under our hijabs.

Whether you're a natural, relaxed, texlaxed, or a transitioning hair sister, this book is for you. Your hair textures may not be the same, but our struggle of maintaining a healthy head of hair under the hijab is same.

With your dedication, patience, and positive intentions, you can gain healthier, stronger, and hijab-friendly hair, insha'Allah.

Let's get you started on the journey.

Bismillah!

What Does Your Hair Mean To You?

Everyone has their personal definition of what they feel their hair means to them, and I know it can mean a variety of things, depending on your mood, social status, financial status, the time of the month, and whether you've just delivered a baby or are entering menopause.

Your hair could mean a head of hair that is protected with your hijab from elements such as pollution and weather, yet it's damaged by the lack of time, knowledge, and commitment to looking after and maintaining a healthy and beautiful head of hair.

Does it mean how lumpy and bumpy your hijab looks with each and every style you possess? Does it mean the struggle you go through watching video after video, stopping and pausing every couple minutes, imitating every move they make and still your hair doesn't come out looking as flawless as theirs?

Lastly does your interpretation mean that no matter what you do or have done, your hair is a hot mess and you have resulted to constantly wearing head coverings as it's easier to say that you're going through an 'Afrocentric phase' at each and every party?

For me, my hair means all of the above and more, so whether you feel your hair is a hot mess, can't or wont be tamed, understand that its your hair and with time and patience it will be nurtured back to restore its beauty of shine, its character of curls and its royalty in its sway. In my opinion, the beauty of a woman begins with her hair; if my hair is right, then my face and outfit is right, too.

"Allah is beautiful and He loves beauty."

– Sahih Muslim

In Islam, there is so much emphasis on what a woman can and can't do to her hair — from cutting, colouring, and oiling it, to using extra hair and plaiting — that as a revert who came from wearing weaves, braids, and wigs, it left me feeling lost and thinking there was nothing else I can do to my hair. Alhamdulillah (all praises are due to God), we cover and understand the importance of covering, but if you allow me to take you back to those days before hijab, how on point was your hair? How many tubs of gel and grease did you go through to get your desired style? How many times did you sit in the salon waiting for hours on end just to be seen to? How many painful braiding and weaving sessions did you endure? Now you wear hijab, what has changed apart from being a little older, working, studying, or being married with children?

We live in an era where social media plays a big role in how we are as consumers, and we are constantly exposed to the perceived glamour of Brazilian, Peruvian, and Indian hair and the never ending kinks and curls of weaves and wigs. And because women are faced with the persistent reminder of what social media decides is the next best thing, many women are left feeling low, depressed, and inadequate against photos with the hashtag '#goals'. We are facing testing times when it comes to beauty, fashion, and hair, but I encourage you to remain steadfast and know that you are beautiful, intelligent, creative, loving, brave and worthy of your own admiration and affection, despite the pressure to share all that you possess with the world.

In today's society, it's very important to learn and teach self-love and appreciation, as this is the foundation of a strong, beautiful, and believing woman.

I, too, am guilty when it comes to trolling many social media sites watching video after video, sliding through picture after picture, and still left feeling baffled and deflated as to why my hair never turned out how the girls in those videos and pictures looked.

This is when I realised my hair is unique to me. The way my hair grows and the speed it grows is individual to my DNA; the girl on the screen and I do not possess these two things the same. The way I style, manage, and care for my hair is in the way my hair best responds; once I understood this, the more enjoyable my hair care and styling process became.

Blank Canvas

As Muslims, we believe our bodies and health are a trust from Allah, and we should look after them to the best of our abilities. We are taught self-love before loving others, and this starts with accepting our hair without adding anything to it whether to enhance its beauty or its length.

Nowadays, the internet has an unimaginable amount of information on how and what products we can use on our hair; there are tons of books that break down the science of hair as well as what hair type you are, but none of them address the everyday issues we face as women who cover our hair.

Where I start with all the sisters who come to see me for the first time, whether they are natural or relaxed, is with a blank canvas. What do I mean by this? I like to strip the hair right back and return what I'm sure it has lost through styling, heat, and environmental damage. I do this by starting with a heavy protein treatment and a black tea rinse, and ending it with a moisturising deep conditioning treatment. This process helps me put the hair in a recovering stage and allows me to fully control the amount of love and care it will receive from then on. Not everyone has access to a hair care stylist, so allow me to walk you through this process if you'd also like to reset your hair and start from a fresh blank canvas so you can build your hair regimen.

First, wash your hair using a clarifying shampoo — this removes every ounce of build-up, dirt, and oil on your scalp and hair — then follow this with a heavy protein treatment. This will help replace any lost proteins that have escaped, and is the first step in allowing your hair to absorb moisture and giving it a fresh start to encourage growth.

Moving on to a black tea rinse will help fight against shedding, and it naturally darkens, adds shine, and strengthens the hair as black tea contains caffeine and this helps block a hormone called DHT (Dihydrotestosterone) that is responsible for hair loss. I particularly encourage sisters who are experiencing postnatal shedding to use a black tea rinse at least once a week and no more than once a week as the scalp is absorbing the caffeine and could pass into breast milk. Everybody reacts differently to the use of caffeine, but the last thing anybody wants is a baby coo'ing and ga'ing through the night.

After the strengthening process the last step would be to give your hair a moisturising deep conditioning treatment using a conditioner of your choice. I am a lover of adding oils to hair conditioners to maximise its healing properties, and there are many testimonies from women who have noticed a significant difference in their hair after adding oils into their hair care regimen. Reports ranged from their hair being softer and shinier, to noticing their hair retaining more moisture than before they added oils. Some of my favourite oils and staples in my regimen are: Coconut oil, olive oil, almond oil, black seed oil, and black castor oil. As there is no one size fits, experiment and see what oils become your favourite.

I suggest leaving the moisturising deep conditioner on your hair for at least 20 minutes and sitting under a steamer, steaming cap, or a hooded dryer. If you do not have the option of one of the 3 steaming methods, I suggest leaving the conditioner on your hair with a shower cap for an hour. There are many ways you can achieve a steam if you do not own a hair steamer, for example, having a hot, steamy shower whilst allowing the steam to penetrate your hair shaft beneath the shower cap; or putting your shower cap on and belly dancing (or any other dance move) to work up a sweat, burning calories, and release natural heat from your head. Another option is to wrap a microwaved towel on your head while you read, drink tea, and put your feet up.

After washing out your conditioner, it is only natural to reach for a towel and rub your hair dry because that's what we have always been taught.

But, there is one rule I always obey and will never go back on, and it is I never use a towel to dry my hair; instead, I use a cotton T-shirt to pat my hair dry. This method reduces frizz, reduces split ends, and minimises damage to the overall health of your hair. Give it a go. I promise you will never go back.

The next step is to use a leave-in conditioner, oil, and a moisturising cream of your choice. The order of how you use these products are famously known as the L.O.C. or L.C.O method: L – leave-in conditioner, O – oil, and C – cream moisturiser, such as the Shea mix in the DIY chapter. The L.C.O. method uses the cream before the oil. These methods use each product to seal the previous one in, to reduce the amount of moisture loss you experience during the day. Have a go at using both methods to see which one works best for your hair. Be open to do things differently and know that if your hair doesn't like something you use or the technique you use, you will be the first to know as your hair will show in the way it feels and looks.

Once you hair is washed, conditioned, and moisturised, there are 2 ways you can dry your hair. You can either blow dry, or air-dry your hair. If you are going to blow dry it, be sure to use a heat protectant and set the blow dryer on medium or low heat. Air-drying is simply leaving your hair to dry using no heat appliances; instead, you use good old fresh air until your hair becomes completely dry. Some women use this method for convenience as well as a healthier way to keep their hair from becoming heat damaged. Remember, there isn't a right or wrong way to go about it, just what works for you. It's your hair, your journey, and only you can know what's good for the health of your hair, or what is just convenient.

This process is straightforward, and although it requires time and effort, the satisfaction of seeing your hair in a healthier condition is definitely worth it.

Cue, hair flick!

Ghusl and Your Hair

Growing up as a black girl in the UK, there were many taboos I was brought up with, especially when it came to the subject of water and my hair. As far back as I can remember, the first thing I did when it rained was to cover my hair, and I never dared to dip my hair in the water when I frequented swimming pools.

Islam emphasises the use of water, as it is our primary source of purification; so that involves getting our hair wet — a lot. As a revert, going from a background where I never wet my hair, to wetting my hair at least 5 times a day to make wudu — or the number of times one can make ghusl in a single day, as newlyweds may attest to — my mind went in to overdrive with all sorts of thoughts. 'Wet my hair 5 times a day?', 'I'm going to walk around with wet hair?', 'But I've just relaxed my hair, though!' — I'm sure you've had those thoughts at some point, too.

There are many misconceptions when it comes to water and the usage of it in our hair, but truth be told, our hair is like a seed: Once planted, keep watering it and it will flourish and grow. Unlike a plant, we can never use too much water in our hair, as it helps seal in moisture, keeps your scalp healthy, and supports your hair growth.

Unlike wudu, ghusl is the ritual bath we have to purify ourselves in preparation for prayer and worship in two circumstances: After our monthly periods, and after what a good friend of mine calls 'va va vroom time'. Both of these baths require getting our hair wet monthly, if not at least twice a week. Wetting our hair on a monthly basis after a period is easy to do and can be manageable, but doing this more than a few times a month can leave us in the dark on how we can further manage a healthy head of hair that's frequently drenched.

As a newlywed, the thought of wetting our hair several times a week can be worrying, especially for sisters with relaxed hair. In desperation, many forcibly embrace their natural hair as last resort to 'save' it from unimaginable breakage and damage. To add to that, friends whose hair has suffered damage from the constant drowning in water also advise them to turn natural. Now, I'm not here to dissuade you from being natural if that's a choice you wish to make, but I'm assuring you that whether you are rocking your natural curls or you have a crown of relaxed hair, ghusl can be something you enjoy from va va vroom all the way to the bath.

As there are two ways for ghusl to be performed, there will be a slightly different method on the care of your hair for each one. These methods are not defined by the texture or type of hair you have, so both relaxed-haired and natural-haired sisters can use these methods.

Ghusl for Intimacy

Before you start your bath after intimacy, if your hair is in braids then just go ahead and make ghusl – if your hair is loose then the first thing to do is to detangle your hair. I advise using a detangling spray or a spritz of water and oil to melt those tangles away. When you are using the oil to help detangle, be sure not to use too much, as we know that oil can create a barrier from the water being absorbed — a condition for valid ghusl — so light usage will be enough to keep your hair moisturised without creating a barrier.

Either finger detangle, or use a wide-tooth comb to detangle your hair. Following detangling, lightly moisturise your hair with a cream and finish off with sealing in the moisture with a light oil such as almond, jojoba, or coconut oil. What this does is prepare your hair to seal in the moisture further with the water you will use on your hair, as the water allows penetration of each layer of product as well keeping your hair moisturised whilst air drying or blow drying.

Ghusl for Menses and Post-Partum Bleeding

The second method of ghusl is performed when you have finished your menses or post-natal bleeding, and has a single difference in how you wash your hair, based on a hadith found in Sahih Bukhari & Muslim where Umm Salamah (may Allah be pleased with her) reported she said to Rasulullah, "O Allah's messenger! I am a woman who tightly braids my hair. Should I unbraid it for the ghusl janabah?" He replied: "No. It would suffice you to pour over your head three cups of water, and then spread the water over the rest of your body – that would make you clean."

This hadith clearly mentions the ghusl of intimacy, thus implying that you have to take down your braids for the ghusl of menses and post-partum bleeding. Thus I would advise you to take advantage of this time to make use of a clarifying shampoo as well as a protein conditioner. Follow the steps I laid out in the Blank Canvas chapter, and give your hair a deep cleansing and a deep conditioning reset. I see this bath as an opportunity to restart our hygiene and beauty routines, and I like to really capitalise on this time of the month to reset and offer myself some pampering time, which is in line with the Sunnah of the Prophet (saw) who timed us to clip our nails and remove all body hair every 40 days.

The overall aim of following these methods is to minimalise dry hair and keep your hair moisturised without compromising the health of your hair, which will allow your hair to thrive and grow.

So, who's ready to make ghusl?

Night-Time Routine

At night, your hair and pillow tend to have a friction fight. As we move around in bed, our hair suffers from damage which leaves us with split ends, breakage, and loss of moisture.

Understandably, after covering your hair with a hijab all day, who wants to cover up again at night? And then you have to deal with the sighs, groaning, and moaning from the husband who detests your satin bonnet and throws shady comments to deter you from wearing it. And what about feeling sick and tired of waking up in the middle of the night to find your bonnet on the floor or under you in the sheets?

In Islam, we are taught to beautify ourselves for our husbands and visa versa, but the night-time bonnet has you conflicted as you have read many articles that basically say either cover your hair with the satin bonnet, or face having damaged and dry hair.

I have a few tips for you to avoid the husband groans and the waking up to find the bonnet elsewhere, and still maintain a healthy head of hair and enjoy sleeping without the bonnet. In order for these tips to work, you need to get into a habit of taking some time each night, or at least every other night to make it work. Life and commitments can play a part in us sometimes cutting corners — and yes, it will happen occasionally — but if you are making the effort 80% of the time, the 20% when you cut corners will not drastically affect the health of your hair.

Before going to bed or whilst you are sitting up in bed, follow the L.O.C or L.C.O method as mentioned in the Blank Canvas chapter. At night, whilst we are asleep, our bodies go into repairing mode and will draw from all sources to take in moisture. It primarily starts with our hair, so if you do not follow the moisturising method and you do not cover your hair with a satin bonnet, you will wake up with dry coarse feeling hair.

If you are planning a braid or twist out for the following day, then now would be a good time to put in your braids or twists. For the natural-haired sisters, I suggest you do this anyway to keep your hair from becoming tangled, as it will reduce your detangling session on your next wash.

Once you have moisturised and sealed your hair, tie your hair up in a loose bun at the top of your head. This is known as the pineapple, and will keep your ends tucked away and protected from being snapped in a way that causes split ends, and will keep your hair moisturised.

The last step to keep your hair and bed a bonnet-free zone is to splash some cash on satin or silk pillowcases. Satin and silk are both known to be gentle on the hair, and allow your hair to retain moisture. While this is a great way to avoid wearing a bonnet at night, I must warn you that sleeping on satin and silk in the summer can be sweaty, so I personally choose to use a satin bonnet and a normal pillowcase during warmer months.

Using these tips will give you a much-needed treat with beautiful satin or silk pillowcases, keep away the husband grumble, and help you sleep like a princess knowing your hair is protected throughout the night.

Hair Typing

'Hair typing' is something my natural-haired sisters may have come across, or may be something you have never heard of. Put simply, it's a method that some swear by and many others have abandoned.

The hair-typing system was created by Andre Walker, Oprah Winfrey's hair stylist of over 25 years and is a way to classify the different curls and sizes natural hair can come in. While there are many hair-typing systems out there, Andre Walker's is the most popular and widely used system in the world.

Please see the chart below for all the different hair types.

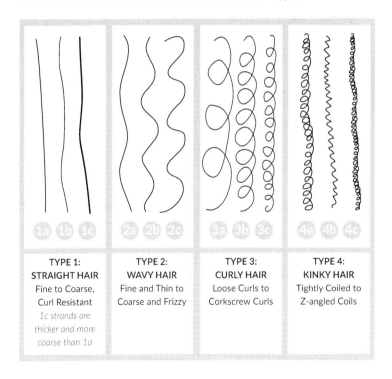

TYPE 1: STRAIGHT HAIR	TYPE 2: WAVY HAIR	TYPE 3: CURLY HAIR	TYPE 4: KINKY HAIR
Fine to Coarse, Curl Resistant	Fine and Thin to Coarse and Frizzy	Loose Curls to Corkscrew Curls	Tightly Coiled to Z-angled Coils
1c strands are thicker and more coarse than 1a			

Those who follow hair-typing rules will tell you that the products you should use in your hair will differ, and the types of styles you should consider might not be right for your hair type. Personally, I do not follow any type of hair typing, for the reasons I share below.

1. Hair typing hurts our community as black women. Within the natural hair community, some women feel bullied and isolated, leading to them disliking their hair, which is the opposite of what Allah wants for us.

2. Hair typing is not a reliable way to determine the health of your hair, nor does it mean that your hair is healthier than other women with different hair types.

3. Most women will find that they may have up to 3 different types in their hair, leading to possible conflicts in how they're told is the 'best' way to care for the different hair types.

4. I have always been of the opinion that when a woman embraces her natural hair, she is also embracing herself in her natural form. Allah created us all in different ways, and we are taught to love ourselves in the same way.

I am a big believer in the fact that it's not what products you use, rather it's the way in which you use the products that will prove most effective. The aim is to achieve healthy hair by equipping yourself with the right knowledge so you gain healthy hair and length, too.

Co-Wash vs. Shampoo

You may have heard of many sisters using the term 'co-washing', but what is co-washing?

Co-washing is simply washing your hair using a conditioner rather than a shampoo.

As shampoo is a cleanser, it can strip your hair of moisture and leave your hair feeling dry, rough, and squeaky clean, depending on the type of shampoo and the ingredients. What's wrong with your hair being squeaky clean? Absolutely nothing once or twice a month, but the constant stripping can lead to damaged hair, especially during the warmer months.

A co-wash is excellent to use during the warmer weather months, on holiday, after a workout, or to alternate between washes. The main use of a co-wash is to put moisture back in your hair whilst cleaning it at the same time. As it is a conditioner, it is important to note that if you co-wash regularly, you are guaranteed to have product build-up, so you will have to make sure that at least once every 4 weeks you use a clarifying shampoo to rid your hair and scalp of the build-up.

Co-washing your hair is an excellent way of cleansing your hair, but I often see many sisters use this method alongside a deep moisturising conditioning treatment. Doing this can lead to your hair becoming over-moisturised, which in turn can lead to breakage and damage. A co-wash is when your hair needs a quick moisture fix.

My natural sisters, a co-wash is a brilliant way of achieving a moisture boost for ghusl, before a braid and twist out, before a spontaneous night in with your girls or the hubby, or whenever your hair feels it needs a quick little pick-me-up.

Sisters who are relaxed can definitely benefit from using co-washes, just as the natural sisters all of the above applies to you too. With relaxed hair, just be sure to also use your protein conditioners as well as the moisturising conditioners, as using too much moisture can quickly lead to moisture overload.

Co-Wash Pros

• Allows the hair and scalp's natural oils to aid in the cleansing of the hair

• Conditioners are water-based, which aids the hydration of your hair

• Helps reduce tangles and knots

• Great for giving the scalp a moisture boost

Co-Wash Cons

• Leaves product build up if used too often
• Hair can become over-moisturised
• The need to wash your hair more often in order to keep a clean and dirt-free scalp.

Styling

Being a natural, transitioning, or texlaxed sister has its moments when it comes to styling your hair, especially under the hijab. If it goes well, then you end up with either bouncy, juicy twists/braids, or perfected flat twist. Maybe those edges are laid and are behaving, or you finally managed to tie your hair back into a hair band in less than 5 minutes.

Now we all know that sometimes our hair has a vibrant personality of its own, not always wanting to be tamed or laid down. With a personality as big as our curls, who would want to be tamed and laid every day, but our hijab requires a level of obedience from our tresses.

Many sisters have succeeded in finding what works for them, and some are still on a journey of trial and error, which is a good thing as you find out what works for you and your hair. For those of you who are still searching for what works, I have a few styles you could use to see what works for you.

Flat Twists

For those of us old enough to know, flat twists are not a new concept of protective hair styling. I candidly remember the times I would sit during my lunch break with a tub of gel and my friend flat twisting my hair. I would change the style of flat twist, weekly, ranging from half-head, full-head, and quarter-head flat twists along with rubber bands to secure them.

Flat twists, for me, are more preferable than cornrows as they are easier on the hair line and they are not tight on the scalp. The best thing about flat twists is they are a great style to wear under the hijab, as they lay flat against the scalp and allow the hijab to lay flat, too.

Cornrows

Cornrows will always be a popular choice, as many of us have culturally grown up using this method as a default for protective styling. My advice to you would be not to only use this method to style your hair. As pretty as they can look, they do have their downfalls, which I list below.

1. Thinning edges – This can occur when the hair is constantly pulled around the edges to achieve a particular style, which can be worsened with the tightness of the hijab or under scarves.

2. Hair loss – Hair loss can happen at any time, especially as we age, but the taking down of cornrow styles can cause hair loss in spots and all over the head.

3. Thinning hair – This is caused by stressing the hair when 'installing' and taking down cornrows.

What can you do to minimise these downfalls? Space out how often you cornrow your hair — with a 1 to 2-week gap before you put them in again; change the style often; ask the stylist to be gentle on your scalp; and lastly, be bold in letting your stylist know that you want her to be easy on your edges.

When taking down cornrows, I recommend that you give it a day before you wash and condition. Taking down hair from a style is a stressful time for your hair; the pulling, tugging, and combing cause damage if not done in the correct way. Remember that because your hair had been in a protective style, naturally shed hair will come away when taking the style down; so do not be alarmed when your comb fills up with hair. When your comb collects an amount that is more than what you are used to, this is a sign that your hair is shedding and/or breaking due to damage caused.

Single Twists and Plaits

Singles are a perfect way of giving your hair a break from the pulling and tugging back cornrows do, but you can still come across the same issues when tying your twists or plaits back to put your hijab on. Here are few suggestions that may alleviate the pulling back of hair before wearing your hijab.

1. Loosen the plaits around your hair line

2. Regularly change your parting when tying your hair back

3. Wear your hair down under your hijab, if you're comfortable with it, as this would give your hair line and scalp the much needed break from constantly being tied back.

Yarn (Wool) Braids and Twists

Using yarn or wool to style hair has been used for many years within many cultures. As wool is a fabric, it is a healthier option compared to using synthetic or human hair. Wool helps the hair retain moisture; it's light on the hair; and can help you achieve many styles.

Just as with any protective style, be sure to regularly keep your hair moisturised either by using a water and oil mix, or using a shop-bought moisturising spray. All protective styles ideally should be worn for a maximum of 4 weeks, with a minimum of a 1-week break before the next protective style.

Bantu Knots

Bantu knots are a beautiful way to curl the hair without the use of excessive heat; you can achieve bouncy curls regardless of the texture of your hair.

When using Bantu knots to achieve a define curl pattern, many sisters are often dissatisfied with the results, especially on the day or night of a party, date night, or a girls' night in. This is something I have learnt the hard way, too, but I soon noticed where I and many other sisters are going wrong.

To achieve a really good Bantu knot out, always give your hair enough time to dry, whether you wash it first, or you start on dry hair and use products to set the Bantu knots. If you are pressed for time, the next best thing to do is to sit under a hooded dryer or use a hair dryer to completely dry the hair. Drying the hair allows the hair to set; you can then continue to leave in the knots so you can get tighter, bouncier, and more defined curls.

Twist Outs

Twists outs are another way of curling your hair without the use of excessive heat. Twist outs give you a different pattern of curl from the Bantu knot out curl. Twist outs are extremely popular, and more commonly used because of the versatility of the twists while you have them in before the take down.

Just as the Bantu knots are put in either wet or dry, always allow sufficient time for twists to dry. Ensuring that your hair is completely dry is crucial to how the curls take in your hair. If you are pushed for time, use a hooded dryer or hair dryer, and then take down the twists either immediately or when you have reached your venue.

I am often asked how to wear twist outs and Bantu knot outs when going to a party, and how to wear the hijab over it. My advice is to take down the twists or knots with a light oil and do not separate. Wear a satin bonnet in order to keep the curls from frizzing. To keep the curls from dropping, a satin bonnet will be your best friend rather than a satin scarf. When you arrive at your venue, take out your hair from the bonnet and separate the curls, fluff, and off you go.

Taking Down Protective Styles

When taking down any protective style, it's important that you be gentle and patient. Although you used the style as a means to better the health of your hair, the take down can undo all that work.

There is a method I always advise sisters to follow when taking down protective styles, and while it does take a little longer than what you might be used to, you are preserving the health of your hair in the long term. In time, and as you get more familiar with the routine, you will get quicker, and I am sure you will find little ways to make it an easier and better routine for yourself.

Before taking down a protective style, I suggest spritzing your hair with water and oil, or a shop-bought detangling spray. What this does is dampens the hair whilst adding a little moisture, and will ensure that snags or knots can gently melt away.

Rub a little coconut oil or an oil of your choice between your fingers and start to take out the braids, twists, or whatever style you have. Using your fingers will reduce the damage to your ends and is so much gentler on your hair. Once all the hair is out, spritz the hair again and divide into four sections.

Mix a cheap conditioner with some oils and apply to each section. For natural, texlaxed, transitioning, and sisters who are stretching their relaxer, I would advise finger detangling once all the conditioner has been applied in your hair. For relaxed-hair sisters and those with minimal regrowth, you may want to use a wide-tooth comb to detangle. This part is just to detangle and get your hair knot-free before washing it. When you are finally ready to wash your hair, it will be tangle-free, soft, and moisturised.

Relaxing and Texlaxing the Right Way

Despite many sisters choosing to embrace their natural hair, there are still many who choose to relax their hair. Whatever your reasons are, I am here to support you by equipping you with the right knowledge on how to best achieve healthy relaxed hair.

There are two ways relaxed-hair women retouch their hair: Relaxing until their hair is bone-straight, or relaxing the hair while leaving some texture – this is what we call texlax. Some say texlaxing your hair is a better option, as you are not completely breaking down the protein bonds in your hair, which results in hair that is thicker and healthier than a bone straight relaxer.

Many sisters have never have attempted to relax or texlax their own hair, and have always entrusted this process to either a hair salon or a family member. In many instances, the method used to process their hair has been wrong; leaving the hair over-processed, and left scalp sore and burnt.

Now, there is nothing wrong with imploring someone else to put relaxer in your hair, but it's vital that you tell them how you want it done. If you are getting a retouch done, let the stylist know that you only want relaxer on the new growth not from root to tip. If you do decide to take control and relax yourself, but feel afraid to do it or just didn't know where to start, I have a few tips that will keep your relaxed and texlaxed hair in tip-top shape.

The process of relaxing your hair should always start from a week before the relaxer is due, and helps to prep and protect your hair through the relaxing process and beyond.

So let's have countdown to your next relaxer or texlaxer date.

Day 1

Detangle and wash your hair with a clarifying shampoo. Remember, this shampoo is like the reset wash for your hair as it completely removes all build in your hair as well as your scalp. The number of times you wash it is entirely up to you, although I like to do things in 3s.

I know you may have raised your eyebrows or even kissed your teeth at the thought of washing your hair before relaxing it because we have all been brought up with the notion that relaxing your hair whilst dirty is better, but I can firmly say this is just misinformation our parents were raised with.

Once you have washed your hair, the next step is to use a strong protein conditioner. I always suggest using Aphogee as it is what has worked best for me and other sisters I have used it on. There are many other brands, so please do your research and find what works best for you. You will notice that when you wash out the protein, your hair will be somewhat hard and dry, yet it will feel strong. This is normal, and is proof that your hair has taken the protein well.

When you have washed out the strong protein conditioner, you will need to use a deep moisturising conditioner — this will put the moisture back in your hair. I love mixing oils and conditioner together to maximise healing properties. Apply the conditioner and use a steamer or a hooded dryer if you have access to either of them, as gentle heat helps the conditioner and oils penetrate your hair further by swelling the hair shaft, opening the cuticles, and allowing your strands to hold more moisture. Once done, use your leave-ins, oils, and moisturising cream, as usual.

Days 6, 5, 4, and 3

As Muslim women, our hair will inevitably get wet whether through ghusl or wudu. Unfortunately, it can be tough to have hair that is fully dry before chemical treating it, however, it's important you keep your hair moisturised by lightly oiling it, as well as comb and itch-free.

Day 2

Part your hair into 4 sections and base your scalp with petroleum jelly (i.e. Vaseline). Oil the already relaxed parts of your hair to keep them safe in the event that the relaxer gets onto them.

Relaxer Day

If you are going to the salon, then you have prepared your hair from any damage that either the relaxer or bad practice from the stylist can cause.

If you have decided to take on this task of doing it yourself: Congratulations! After you self-relax for the first time, you will feel liberated and will ask yourself why you used to pay someone to do it for you. I must advise that you ensure you are fully prepared with everything you need right beside you. If you have children and are able to have them entertained during this time, that's perfect; if not, I advise you to wait for them to get to 'lala land' before you start.

Once you have chosen the right time to relax or texlax your hair, follow these steps to help you relax and texlax the right way:

Step 1 – Part your hair into 4 sections.

Step 2 – Base your hairline with Vaseline – you can never base your edges too much.

Step 3 – Mix the activator with the relaxer. I always add 2-4 tablespoons of coconut or castor oil to the mix, too, as it helps weaken the relaxer slightly, which gives you a shiny and moisturised finish.

Step 4 – Apply the mixture to your new growth. I always suggest starting from the part of your hair that takes longest to take to the relaxer; in my case, it is the back of my head. Work through each section and apply the relaxer. You may ask about using a comb to stretch the relaxer through the new growth. This is optional, as I know some women like the bone-straight look. Personally, I don't stretch the relaxer through the new growth as I feel it over-stresses the hair. The alternative to this would be to use your fingers to smooth the new growth out.

If you are not confident in doing the whole head all at once, that's fine. Go ahead and wash out the relaxer from the part that you had relaxed first, whilst not getting the part you have not relaxed wet.

Step 5 – Wash out the relaxer, apply your protein-based deep conditioner, and complete the last step by using a neutralising shampoo.

I always apply a deep conditioner before the shampoo in order to to rebuild the protein bonds the relaxer broke down. If you are not self-relaxing, be firm in asking your stylist to do this for you. Some stylists will probably charge extra and roll their eyes, or tell you that you 'can't do this', so go equipped with your own protein-based deep conditioner.

For those who wish to leave some texture in their hair instead of the bone-straight relax, all of the above applies to you, too, the only difference is the length of time the relaxer is left in your hair; it would be shorter and does not require the smoothing out process.

While it may seem daunting at first, I promise the relaxer process outlined above will get easier and faster with each and every application, and I guarantee that you will have a healthier head of relaxed hair as a result, insha'Allah. Use it as a time to give your hair the special works and you will be able to enjoy the sway and 'I'm worth it' moments as you keep it moisturised and nourished with what it needs when it needs it.

Shedding, Breakage, & Split Ends

Shedding is a natural process our hair goes through. Throughout our life, the shedding process can either speed up or slow down. Times when shedding speeds up could be due to many changes the body may be going through, such as pregnancy, breastfeeding, hormonal imbalances and changes, vitamin deficiencies, illness, and ageing.

These contributing factors will vary from woman to woman, but most of us will have experienced excessive shedding at some point within our life. If dealt with properly, the shedding will slow down and resume to its normal shedding rate; but if care is not taken, the excessive shedding will turn to breakage.

How do you know if your shedding is normal? The answer to this question will differ for all women, but now would be a good time to start noticing how much you shed on an everyday basis. Run your comb through your hair and see how much hair you have on your comb, use this as a basis and manage your shedding from here on out.

Hair breakage can be a stressful occurrence to deal with; every time you comb your hair, run your fingers through or even simply take your hair down from a protective style, you see hair all over the floor. Breakage usually happens because the hair is lacking something; maybe you overloaded it with moisture or protein, or you used a product your hair didn't like; maybe it's lacking moisture or protein, or it could be that your hair needs a little love from you.

Split ends are easy to go unnoticed, but they are more common than most people think. They appear at the very end of a hair strand and look 'split'. Many women will ask, 'How do I get split ends?' For some women it's heat, colour, or chemical damage, and for others it's lack of proper care on a daily basis; but the simplest of it is split ends can just happen.

If split ends occur and are not treated, they can split further up the hair strand and damage it, which leads to breakage. Despite claims that you can heal split ends, the reality is you can't. Once strands have split, the only way to treat them is to trim off the split ends and avoid what caused them to split in the first place. You may feel split ends are not a big deal, however, they are. Split ends can hinder hair growth and set you back in your hair journey.

What does breakage look like?

Breaking hair is very distinct and you will very quickly know that your hair is suffering from breakage as the breaking hair will be many in number and look like little cut pieces of hair.

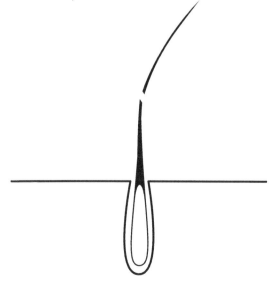

What does shed hair look like?

Shed hair are strands you see on your comb; one end will have a white bulb, which shows the life cycle of the hair has been complete and has fallen from the follicle.

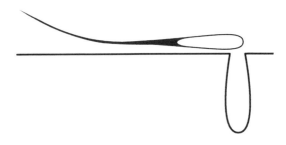

How can you slow down excessive shedding?

As I outlined in the Blank Canvas chapter, a black tea rinse is an excellent way of bringing hair shedding back down to its normal rate. Black tea contains a block hormone called DHT, which helps slow down shedding. It's always a good idea to use a black tea rinse at least once every 6 weeks as a preventative measure.

How can you stop breakage?

The first step is to establish what is causing your breakage, then you can start to nurture your hair back to a healthier state. I would strongly suggest you follow the Blank Canvas treatment and then follow up with weekly deep conditioning treatments.

How can I manage split ends?

Every 6 weeks I give my hair a mini trim and I advise you do the same. There are many videos online that can walk you through the process of mini trims. It's best to keep heat to a minimum; if your hair is colour-treated, ensure you keep up with your weekly treatments to keep dryness at bay. Always pay attention to your ends when moisturising and sealing as they are the oldest parts of your hair and will need the most care, compared to the new growth coming from your scalp.

Moisture & Protein Overload

Moisture and protein overload are very common, and most of the time you won't realise you have done this to your hair. When the hair is overloaded, it starts to feel different, look unusual, and becomes hard to manage. Both natural and relaxed hair can fall victim to a moisture and protein overload, although chemically-treated hair is at a higher risk of protein overload than non chemically-treated hair.

In our quest to keep our hair moisturised and strong with protein treatments, we can overdo it, which ultimately leads to not just hair damage, but also distress to yourself as you may not know what to do. You need to be sure that you alternate between moisturising your hair and giving it protein treatments as and when it needs it. The key is to listen to what your hair needs rather than what you want to give it, and you'll generally know what it needs by how it feels.

Moisture Overload

If your hair is overloaded with moisture, it will feel gummy or mushy when it's wet, which is an indication that your hair needs a protein-based conditioner to help counteract the moisture. After this, you should alternate between moisturising and using protein conditioners, and avoid overnight deep conditioning and over-moisturising your hair.

Protein Overload

Protein overload can sometimes be hard to tell just by the feel or look of your hair because dry hair and protein-overloaded hair look and feel the same. Your hair will feel dry and brittle, no matter how many times you moisturise it. The best way to know if you have protein overload is to do a strand elasticity test while your hair is wet, which is best to do whilst washing your hair. To do a strand elasticity test, simply pull a strand of hair from each section until it snaps; if you are protein overloaded, then it won't have much of a stretch and will snap quite easily. Why do you need to pull a strand to see how soon it snaps? Protein overload robs your hair of its elasticity, making it more difficult to manipulate and style.

Protein Conditioners Basics

There are 4 types of protein conditioner treatments: protein packs, reconstructors, deep penetrating treatments, and light protein treatments. Depending on the condition of your hair will depend on the type of protein conditioner you will need to use.

For severely damaged hair, you will need to use a reconstructor e.g. Aphogee 2 Min. Reconstructor, or Affirm 5 in 1. Moderate damage uses a deep-penetrating conditioner e.g. ORS Hair Mayonnaise, or Aphogee 2-Step Protein Treatment. For slightly damaged or routine treatments, use light protein treatments e.g. Motions CPR or protein packs such as Palmers Protein Pack.

What can you do to treat moisture overload?

• Wash your hair with a protein shampoo
• Condition your hair with a protein conditioner
• Follow the protein conditioner with a moisturising conditioner
• Use a protein leave-in conditioner
• Follow the LOC or LCO method, then style

I suggest you follow this treatment for at least 3 weeks, then go back to alternating between your moisturising and protein treatments.

What can you do to treat protein overload?

- Wash your hair with a moisturising shampoo
- Condition your hair with a moisturising conditioner
- Use a moisturising leave-in conditioner
- Follow the LOC or LCO method, then style

I suggest you follow this treatment for at least 3 weeks, then go back to alternating between your protein and moisturising treatments.

Underscarves & Hijabs

Wearing our hijab is, of course, a religious obligation, but if worn incorrectly, it can cause a lot of damage to our hair. I guess you're thinking, 'Well, I have to wear hijab, so there's no way around it'. Well, lady, there are ways you can minimise and/or stop hair damage altogether.

Fortunately, we live in a time where hijabs are plentiful in our markets, shops, and bazaars, varying in colour, width, length and material. What's so bad about having these options? Absolutely nothing, apart from the material that some hijabs are made from. In the Night-Time Routine chapter, I spoke about how our pillow absorbs moisture from our hair, and this applies to hijabs in the same way. As beautiful as they may look and make you feel, moisture, frizz, and split ends can become your reality if precaution is not taken whilst wearing your hijab.

Unfortunately, there is no shortcut around protecting your hair when wearing your hijab, but if you follow the adjustments below, your hair will be in better condition all day.

1st – Wear a silk or satin underscarf. This is imperative as it combats frizz, protects your ends from splitting, and keeps moisture locked in. How you wear your underscarf is entirely up to you, just ensure that it covers your hair and ends.

2nd – Change the side of your parting regularly. This will help keep bald patches around your edges at bay.

$3rd$ – Invest in silk or satin hijabs if you just don't want to wear something extra on your hair.

$4th$ – If you feel your hair needs a bit of moisture, spritz with a conditioner and water mixture, then follow up with a light oil. Ensure you wait a while for your hair to dry before wearing your underscarf to avoid the damp musky smell that can occur.

Both natural and relaxed-haired sisters occasionally struggle with unruly edges, but this method will ensure edges are smoothly laid.

Pregnancy Hair

Pregnancy is an exciting time for many women, and a time when women should be in optimal health. Pregnancy books and magazines will tell you how much your hair will grow and glow; how much thicker your hair will become; and how stronger it will feel. Yes, this will be the case for many women, but on the other hand, there are women who experience the exact opposite of all this wonderful stuff that happens when a woman is pregnant.

As much as pregnancy can be a beautiful experience for a woman, it is also a testing time for a woman's body. The baby relies on the mother for protection, nutrients, comfort, and growth. This demand takes everything from what the woman had prior to the pregnancy, and the biggest toll will be taken on by her hair, skin, and nails.

During pregnancy, some women will experience excessive shedding, breakage, and thinning edges, as well as a total loss of edges and hair. Most symptoms only last the duration of the pregnancy, whilst some will continue for at least 9 months after giving birth, and a few will last well into a year post-birth.

The body will do what it naturally wants to do no matter what you do to try and stop it; there are no miracle growth creams, oils, or mixes that will stop the hair going through its natural phase of shedding or breakage whether it's related to hormonal imbalances or not.

Keep up with your weekly deep conditioning with heat, co-washes, moisturising routine. If you are consistent before pregnancy and throughout your pregnancy, the post-birth damage will be minimal; and if there is damage, it will end quickly and you will easily be able to nurture your hair back to its pre-pregnancy state.

Unfortunately, there are no definitive rules when it comes to dealing with pregnancy and hair, so it's best to pay close attention to your hair's needs.

Supplements & Vitamins

I am often asked about the different types of supplements and vitamins that are available — if they are ok to use, whether they help hair grow, and if they are worth the money.

In my personal opinion, what you get from supplements and vitamins you can eat through your food, smoothies, and superfood. Good health always starts from the inside, which will then start to show on the outside, and this applies to good hair health, too. When you look at the market and the various types of hair supplements, there are many to choose from and different prices, and they all ultimately claim to give you healthy, long, strong hair.

When searching for supplements and vitamins to give your hair a book, it's important that you do your research into what ingredients they use, and read reviews from genuine buyers rather than paid reviews or blogger collaborations.

Here are few supplements that are known to support healthy hair growth:

- Hair, skin and nails supplement
- Biotin
- Hairfinity
- Mielle Organics
- The Mane Choice
- Hydratherma

All in all, they are worth a try and your body and hair can only benefit from the extra goodness they give — who doesn't want shiny hair and glowing skin? While supplementing your diet with supplements and vitamins can be beneficial, it's still a good idea to aim to get most of your nutrients from your diet. How you do this, is entirely up to you.

Our body is always repairing itself and will be at its most optimum when we are consuming the right things as well as allowing the body to expel the toxins by exercising. I am not saying you need to embark on a journey of weight loss and become a fitness guru – although that could be beneficial for you – I am advising you that even the bare minimum has brilliant effects on our health, body, and hair.

Some swear by drinking at one green smoothie a day; some say that drinking 8 glasses of water a day keeps you and your hair hydrated; some claim that working out for at least 30 minutes a day will keep the heart healthy. Whilst we do not dispute these claims, we also know that as Muslimahs, we love to enjoy a good meal out, whether it with family or friends, which is fine. Just enjoy in moderation, drink plenty of of water, run with the kids in the park, and do what makes you feel good.

When you look after your health on the inside and on the outside, your body will reward you with healthy hair and glowing skin.

Regimen

In this chapter, you will read other sisters' hair care regimens and what works for them and their hair. No regimen is right or wrong, I have included them as inspiration for you to create a regime that works well for you.

Freshly-relaxed 2 x Weekly Routine

Deep pre-shampoo condition with Philip Kingsley Elasticizer, shampoo with a moisturising shampoo (Aussie, Herbal Essences), and then condition with any moisturising shampoo (Keracare Humecto, Herbal Essences, Cream of Nature).

Post 6 Weeks Relaxer

I leave my hair in conditioner 95% of the time, and will only shampoo my hair if my scalp gets itchy. After every shampoo I use a scalp toner by Philip Kingsley. I always use Mizani milk leave-in conditioner and Mizani butter cream. Sometimes I condition my hair with Amla oil and I'll condition my hair either with Elasticizer or a moisturising conditioner when I feel like my hair is getting dry.

I will comb my hair maybe once, but I'll finger comb every time I condition. I also comb my hair every 2-3 weeks.

Relaxed Hair Regimen

Daily:

Moisturise with ACV (apple cider vinegar), water or aloe juice. Seal with oil or Shea Moisture Jamaican Black Castor Oil (JCBO) styling lotion.

Massage scalp every evening with oil. Sleep on satin pillowcase; use cotton T-shirt to dry hair after washing; use hooded dryer.

Bi-Weekly:
Co-wash, L.O.C. method, and protective style.

Weekly:
Pre-shampoo deep condition with Shea Moisture JCBO treatment mask. Shampoo with Shea Moisture JCBO shampoo, or co-wash depending on level of build-up. L.O.C. method and protective style. Sometimes overnight.

Monthly:
Henna treatment with Lush henna; follow-up with deep conditioning of choice or hot oil treatment. L.O.C method and protective style.

Every 6-12 weeks:
Straighten and trim as necessary.

Natural Hair Regimen
Weekly:
Alternate co-washing with shampooing every other week; deep condition with heat weekly. Black tea rinse with every deep condition; follow the L.O.C method; pull back into a bun, or loosely tie on top of my head if going to bed.

Monthly:
Heavy protein treatment followed by moisturising deep conditioning treatment. L.O.C method; mini trim.

Regimen basics

As you can see from the above regimens, these sisters have found what has worked for them and their hair needs. At the beginning of my healthy hair journey, I sat looking at regimens like these and wondered what I needed to start with.

Below, I have outlined the basics you need in your arsenal — the brands and types are entirely up to you. If you want to channel your inner mixtress then the DIY section would be a good start, too.

Clarifying Shampoo e.g. ORS Aloe Shampoo, or Black African Soap Shampoo from DIY section – use every 4-6 weeks to remove product build-up from the hair and scalp.

Moisturising Shampoo e.g. Crème Of Nature Moisturising Shampoo, or Black African Soap Shampoo from DIY section – use as often as you like during the week or month.

Moisturising Deep Conditioner e.g. Crème Of Nature Orange & Mango Moisturising Deep Conditioner, or Moisturising Deep Conditioner from DIY section – use weekly, alternating with protein conditioners; or used after a reconstructor or deep-penetrating protein treatment.

Protein Deep Conditioner e.g. refer back to the protein basics to determine which protein level your hair may need, or Protein Deep Conditioner from DIY section – use weekly or monthly.

Leave-in Conditioner e.g. Crème Of Nature with Argan Oil Strength & Shine Leave-In Conditioner – use after a wash before using your moisturiser.

Moisturiser e.g. KeraCare Oil Moisturiser with Jojoba Oil, or Shea Butter

Mix from DIY section – use as part of the L.O.C. method.

Oils e.g. coconut oil, olive oil, jojoba oil, argan oil, rapeseed oil, avocado oil, almond oil –Use as part of L.O.C. method.

Co-Wash E.g. Palmers Co-wash or any conditioner of your choice.

DIY Recipes

Hot Oil Treatment

1 teaspoon 100% pure coconut oil
2-3 drops of an essential of your choice
1 teaspoon jojoba oil
1 teaspoon avocado oil
2 tablespoons olive oil

Mix all the ingredients together and heat in the microwave for a few seconds.
Use on your hair as a pre-wash treatment.

Moisturising Deep conditioner

1 tablespoon Shea butter
1 banana
1 teaspoon honey
4 tablespoons mayonnaise
4 tablespoons olive oil
½ cup of natural yoghurt

Blend all ingredients together until smooth. Apply and cover on your hair for
a deep conditioning treatment.

Protein Deep Conditioner

This protein recipe is my favourite. I came across it during one of my
many trolling sessions on YouTube, and it has been my staple ever since.

1 banana
1 cup Aloe Vera Juice
½ can coconut milk
1 tablespoon olive oil
A couple of drops of an essential oil of your choice

Blend all ingredients together until smooth.

Clay Mask treatment

1 cup bentonite clay
2 tablespoons Olive oil
1 tablespoon aloe vera oil or gel
8 drops of an essential oil of your choice
1 cup apple cider vinegar

Mix all ingredients until smooth. Cover the hair with a shower cap or cling film to prevent the mask drying out. Follow up with a moisturising deep conditioner.

Black Soap Shampoo

3 tablespoons crushed black soap
150ml warm water
2 tablespoons olive oil
1 tablespoon vitamin E oil
30 drops of an essential of your choice

Mix and stir all ingredients together. Put aside to allow the soap to melt.

Hair Spritz

Making this spritz has no measurements. I always just go by eye measurements and what seems to feel right.

Water
Conditioner of your choice
Oil of your choice
Optional essential oil of your choice

Henna Treatment

Henna treatments are an excellent way of strengthening and adding shine to the hair, as well covering greys.

200-250g henna
4 tablespoons honey
1 tablespoon black castor oil
1 tablespoon coconut oil
Hot water

Combine ingredients, ensuring you add a little hot water at a time until you get a paste consistency. Ensure you base your edges and ears with Vaseline, as henna will stain if it gets on your skin. I always aim to do a henna treatment at least once every 8 weeks.

Shea Hair Butter Mix

I love using this Shea butter mix in my hair. All hair types would love this butter. You could use as a daily moisturizer, or use it for braids and twist outs. The uses for this butter on your hair, as well as your body, are endless.

250g Shea Butter
1 tablespoon coconut oil
1 tablespoon olive oil
1 tablespoon jojoba oil
1 tablespoon castor oil
30 drops of an essential oil of your choice.

Put water in a pot and bring to the boil. Place the Shea butter in a bowl that can be heated to a high temperature, and place the bowl in the water. Stir the Shea butter until it has melted to an oil consistency. Once it's all melted, take the bowl out of the water and leave to cool. Once cool, add your oil choices.

Put the mix to the side for 30 minutes to allow to cool, and then put the mix in your fridge for an hour.

Take the mix out and whip it until it becomes fluffy. If you want the mix to be more of a balm consistency, do not whip it; simply leave it in the fridge until the mix has set.

28138780R00031

Printed in Great Britain
by Amazon